Substance of Building Healthy Relationships

Barbara Hawkins-Dixon
&
Darlene Mamon

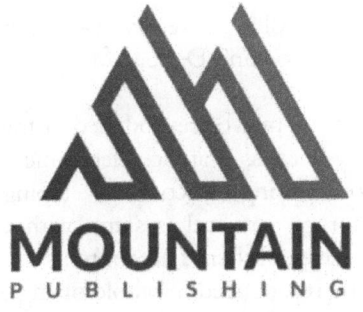

Scripture quotations marked (NKJV) are taken from the New King James Version®. Copyright © 1982 by Thomas Nelson. Used by permission. All rights reserved.

Scripture quotations marked (AMP) are taken from the Amplified Bible, Copyright © 1954, 1958, 1962, 1964, 1965, 1987 by The Lockman Foundation. Used by permission.

Scripture quotations marked (TPT) are from The Passion Translation®. Copyright © 2017, 2018, 2020 by Passion & Fire Ministries, Inc. Used by permission. All rights reserved. ThePassionTranslation.com.

Scripture quotations marked (AMPC) are taken from the Amplified® Bible, Copyright © 1954, 1958, 1962, 1964, 1965, 1987 by The Lockman Foundation. Used by permission. Lockman.org

Scripture quotations marked (MSG) are taken from The Message, copyright © 1993, 2002, 2018 by Eugene H. Peterson. Used by permission of NavPress. All rights reserved. Represented by Tyndale House Publishers.

SUBSTANCE OF BUILDING HEALTHY RELATIONSHIPS

Copyright © 2023 All rights reserved — Barbara Hawkins-Dixon and Darlene Mamon

No part of this book may be reproduced or transmitted in any form or by any means, graphic, electronic, or mechanical, including photocopying, recording, taping, or by an information storage retrieval system without the written permission of the publisher. The contents and cover of this book may not be reproduced in whole or in part in any form without the express written permission of the author or Mountain Publishing.

Please direct all copyright inquiries to:

Mountain Publishing
www.MountainPublishingBooks.com
Phone: (202) 630-5704

Library of Congress Control Number: 2024901260

ISBN (Paperback): 978-0-9991524-5-4
ISBN (Hardback): 978-0-9991524-6-1

Cover and Interior Design: Mountain Publishing Design Team
Editors/Production: Mountain Publishing Production and Editorial Team

Printed in the United States of America

Table of Contents

ENDORSEMENTS I
DEDICATION V
INTRODUCTION 1

CHAPTER 1
SETTING BOUNDARIES 17

CHAPTER 2
THINGS WOMEN AND MEN NEED IN A
RELATIONSHIP 33

CHAPTER 3
TOXIC VERSES HEALTHY 47

CHAPTER 4
IMPORTANCE OF SELF-ESTEEM 59

CHAPTER 5
OVERCOMING ALL OBSTACLES 71

CHAPTER 6
KNOWING YOUR POSITION 81

CHAPTER 7
ACCOMPLISHMENTS AND GOALS 85

CHAPTER 8
NAVIGATING A RELATIONSHIP/CAREER/PARENTING 93

CHAPTER 9
HOW TO BECOME A BETTER PERSON IN THE RELATIONSHIP
.... 99

CHAPTER 10
HOW TO MAKE YOUR RELATIONSHIP SUCCESSFUL 105

GET TO KNOW THE AUTHORS 109

Endorsements

DARLENE MAMON'S CHILDREN:

My mother really has always inspired me, even when I am wrong or make mistakes. She never judges me, and her love remains unconditional, regardless of what I have or have not done. Growing up, I learned how to be respectful and kind to others, even when they are not kind to me by watching her and/or following her lead. My mother's love and guidance has helped to mold me into the man I am today. Her love has always given me the permission and freedom I needed to discover who I am and to live my truth. As a result, this has attracted many people to me. Mere words cannot express my love and appreciation for the woman I call Mom. Just know that every heartbeat reminds me of the sacrifices and the tears she has shed, helping me to love the man looking back at me in the mirror. (Darrius)

A wise woman once said, it is okay to be human. My mother's quiet strength and determination taught me that being strong and having self-discipline prepares you to handle anything life throws your way. Even today I can see her saying, in my mind's eye, do not worry about whether anyone else understands me. Just make sure that I understand myself, my desires, my passion, and my dreams. She is a true Goal Digger. (Jenny)

I learned that giving up and/or giving in is not an option from me. No matter the age, I can make changes and evolve into who I am destined to be. Especially if I am willing to do my personal self-work. I must stay patient and humble and work hard for things to work in my favor. (Tommie)

If there is one word, I can use to describe my mother at this moment, it would be inspirational. Regardless of the circumstances, she has always been there for me, no matter what. My mother continues to push through and make things happen; from her life experiences, creativity, career, and/or continued education. Whatever she puts her mind to, she conquers it. (Tyiasha)

BARBARA HAWKINS-DIXON'S CHILDREN:

Hello, I am Anisha Hawkins, the oldest child and only girl in my family. I feel truly blessed to have such an amazing, inspirational, loving, and strong mother. She has taught me so much about resilience and strength. Anyone to know her would attest to the impact of her strength. I am so proud of my mom and all that she has overcome.

Mom, you rock, and I want you to continue to reach for greatness! I LOVE YOU! (Your One and Only Daughter Anisha)

Hello, I am Joshua Hawkins, and I am the second eldest child. First and foremost, I am beyond grateful that God blessed me with a strong, inspirational, and very talented mother. Hands down, she is the strongest woman I know! Her strength challenges me to be better and to never give up or give in. I'm so proud of you, Mom! LOVE YOU! (Joshua)

Hello, I am Jacki Hawkins, the youngest child of the family. I have been blessed since birth to have a mother like mine. I have watched her go through storms; only to come out better and stronger. I get my strength from her, for sure. I am forever grateful and thankful for your love, support and just being there for me, when I wanted you there and when I didn't. I love you, mom! (Your Youngest Son, Jacki)

Dedication

This book is dedicated to all couples who have experienced or are enduring a toxic relationship. Our aim is to encourage and enlighten you about the warning signs to watch for while dating before entering into a commitment. Drawing from our own experiences with toxic relationships, we have learned that they are fundamentally unhealthy, regardless of appearances. By sharing our struggles, hurts, and pain from past relationships, we hope to offer you insights for your own relationships.

Toxic relationships can erode self-esteem, leaving you feeling at fault for everything. You may question yourself, wondering where things went wrong, even if you did nothing wrong. It is difficult to realize that it is not your fault.

Being in a harmful relationship can lead to health issues like high blood pressure, anxiety, stress, and headaches, along with stomach pains. A toxic relationship often starts by mimicking a healthy one until it doesn't. It can become physically, emotionally, and/or mentally abusive without warning.

Sometimes, we overlook problems in relationships because we are blinded by love, ignoring the warning signs. Many times, we are so attracted to the other person that we have gotten lulled into a false sense of security, and we ignore their personality. We ignore how they represent themselves around others while in our presence.

In marriage, some feel obligated to stay because of the vows they exchanged that committed them "*for better or worse.*" However, these vows do not bind you to a relationship that is harming you from within. They do not justify being treated without love or enduring physical, emotional, or mental abuse. Remember, love is *NOT* supposed to hurt!

Occasionally, we may recognize something is wrong in a relationship but stay, thinking we can change the person. It is critical for couples to understand that people change only when they choose to. Entering a relationship does not mean surrendering your will and/or your ability to live your life as you see fit. Do not shrink as a person to become someone they can accept, because the consequences are too great. Keep in mind, people will do to you only what you allow them to do. You *MUST* learn and accept that you are in control of your life. Regardless of how out of control you may feel your life is, nobody owns you or can be better at being you than YOU!

Life, experiences, and relationships have taught us that before you can truly love anyone else, you must first love yourself. If you have low- self-esteem, you will attract like-minded individuals because like attracts like. Mal Paper says, *"In its simplest form, the law of attraction states that you receive the same energy that you put out into the world."* Meaning, who you see yourself to be on the inside reflects the people you attract into your life. If you secretly hate yourself, that person will privately and publicly treat you like they hate you, and you will allow it because they are mirroring back to you how you feel about yourself.

In every aspect of your life, you must speak up for yourself and use your voice. Relationships are no different. Your voice matters because it speaks to how you demand to be treated and supports the boundaries you set at the beginning of the relationship. Operate within your relationship with integrity. When you speak, say what you mean and mean what you say. Do not let things just happen in the relationship without you voicing your opinion, ideas, needs and/or hurts. Waiting until later is too late for you to voice your concerns while you are simmering underneath about to go off. However, waiting until an appropriate time to have a difficult discussion is always best because it gives you an opportunity to calm down, choose your words wisely, and respect both yourself and the other person.

Remember, the first relationships you are exposed to are within the family unit. If it is dysfunctional and/or abusive, then you have to give yourself permission to learn what a healthy relationship is. You will also have to learn how to love the child within that never received the love they needed to grow and learn how to love themselves. All of this must be done to ensure you can recognize a healthy relationship when it shows up in your life. Being in a healthy relationship offers you peace, joy, contentment, and happiness. So much so that your heart overflows with it. You will know and feel your partner/mate's love, and know you are loved by their actions towards you. It is easy to tell someone that you love them, but their actions towards you will speak louder than their words ever will.

Do not be a willing victim in a toxic relationship. The pain is excruciating and demoralizing. Trust us, we know what it feels like. Do not make the mistake of believing you can handle it and stay longer than you should. The damage from a toxic relationship affects your life, mind, body, and soul. If you are unsure of what is acceptable and unacceptable to maintain a healthy relationship, seek help. We have learned through trial and error, frustration, and pain, and through the trials of our relationships, that toxic relationships leave a bruised and battered version of you behind. That is not what we want for you. We want you to take a page or more out of our book and grow.

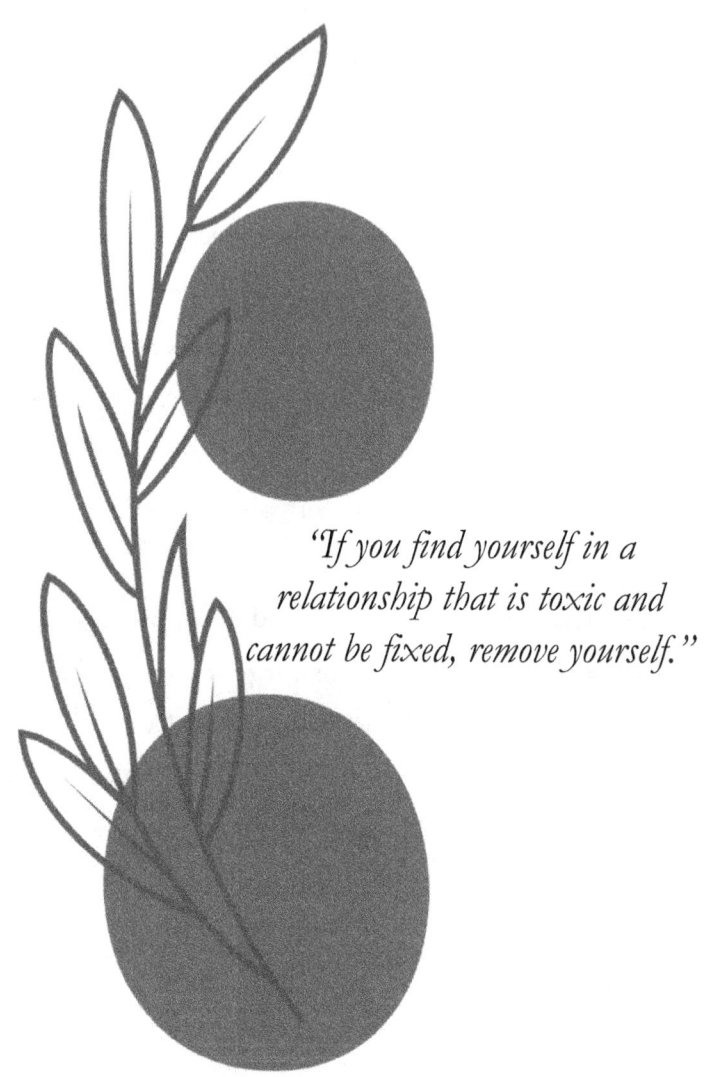

"If you find yourself in a relationship that is toxic and cannot be fixed, remove yourself."

Introduction

Within a relationship, trust, honesty, respect, and communication are fundamental. Traditionally, the man is seen as the provider, and the woman as the help. These roles are rooted in religious texts, such as Genesis 2:18 that says, *"And the Lord God said it is not good that the man should be alone; I will make him and helpmeet for him,"* and 1 Timothy 5:8 states, *"if anyone does not provide for members of his household, he has denied the faith and is worse than an unbeliever."* In today's society, opinions about these roles vary. Some people believe these traditional roles are outdated and should no longer apply. Others argue that the provider's identity in the household is irrelevant, while there are those who maintain that the man should be in control, with the woman playing a subordinate role.

There are even those who believe a woman's place is in the home with the responsibility of taking care of her husband and children, having little involvement in household affairs and business. This view draws on Genesis 2:18, which outlines the role the woman plays in the husband and wife relationship as ordained by God. The word "helpmeet" suggests the woman is there to assist, stepping in where her partner/mate lacks and supporting his efforts. In this context, the roles of the provider and helpmeet are seen as equal; neither the man nor the woman is superior.

However, the challenge arises when these roles are not clearly defined, leaving both partners/mates uncertain of their identities and contributions to the relationship. This uncertainty can lead to a failure of identifying priorities resulting in feelings of neglect, under-appreciation, or undervaluation. It highlights the importance of clear roles and mutual understanding in ensuring the longevity and health of the relationship.

Introduction

POSITIVE ATTITUDE

In any romantic relationship, whether you are married or dating, keeping a positive attitude is essential. Never let your pride override your standards. Setting boundaries early on is important. Clearly define and communicate your do's, don'ts and non-negotiables to your partner/mate. By doing so, you are collectively setting boundaries and/or negotiating the terms of your relationship while building a firm and healthy foundation for your relationship to grow. Otherwise, without such boundaries, a relationship might seem healthy but could be unbalanced, with one partner giving too much and the other taking too much.

If you find yourself in a relationship that is toxic and cannot be fixed, remove yourself. In future relationships, do not repeat past mistakes and leave negative patterns behind. Healing alters your mindset, turning negative self-talk to positivity. This change will be seen in the various aspects of your life, including personal relationships, work and family dynamics.

Substance of Building Healthy Relationships

Understand that men and women often think differently. Men are more logical, analytical, and rational, while women are generally more intuitive, creative, and emotional. Knowing yourself and your needs will help you understand what pleases or upsets your partner/mate.

Relationships are inherently challenging. There will be good days and bad days, but each challenge you face in your relationship does not have to be an insurmountable obstacle. Change begins when you know who you are and your purpose in life. Be realistic about your abilities. Give yourself permission to grow within the relationship and learn more about yourself. As you grow, re-evaluate your do's, don'ts, and non-negotiables, and set standards that support who you are and who you are becoming. This will help you to daily set and attain goals that support the healthy relationship you are building with your spouse/mate.

Ultimately, nurturing healthy relationships contributes to greater happiness.

INTRODUCTION

DEFINING HEALTHY RELATIONSHIPS

Healthy relationships are based on love, respect, trust, and good communication. A healthy relationship is spending quality time with each other, enjoying each other's company, and keeping the flames burning. The connection that you both shared in the beginning should continue to grow, not decrease.

We understand at our age, people need room to change. So, it is important to share your needs, feelings, and thoughts with your mate. As you get older, you might not fulfill your partner/mate's every need or desire; for instance, sex.

SEX IN RELATIONSHIPS

When you are younger in age, sex happens frequently. When you began to gracefully age, some couples do not desire to have sex often. Then there are those who do not even think about sex, and it does not bother them. Understandably, there are couples who do not let their age change their desire for sex. Truth be told, Viagra works when needed (LOL). As we age, some sexual needs or desires are not met because of medical issues. However, what is very important in a healthy relationship/marriage is making sure there is time set aside for quality time and open communication. This will help you and your spouse/mate to talk out and/or work through any obstacles.

TAKE THE PRESSURE OFF

In a healthy relationship, you do not feel pressured into doing anything that is against your will. It is okay to not take part in things that you are not comfortable with. It is important to understand that you both have different needs and desires therefore, each of you should be clear on what the other will or won't do. As you get older, everything you used to do, you may no longer be able to do. Now do not laugh at us, just wait till you become our age. You will see positions will change (LOL). In addition, never agree or get into a habit of doing something that you are not comfortable doing just to please the other

INTRODUCTION

person. It is important that you please yourself as well. If you find yourself pleasing him/her while sacrificing your happiness and/or self-respect, bitterness and resentment may be the result. A result that is felt on the inside and displayed in your treatment of your spouse/mate. In a healthy relationship, you can talk to your spouse/mate about anything without being judged and criticized.

FAMILY IN RELATIONSHIPS

To keep a healthy relationship with your spouse/mate, it is vital to keep family and friends out of your personal business. It can cause strife amongst the family and with friends. Keep in mind that when the two of you decide to forgive each other, many family members are not where you both are. They may still hold animosity towards your mate and aren't capable of or ready to forgive them. They may still cling to a grudge and unforgiveness for what your mate did to you.

In a marriage, never put family or friends before your spouse, not even your mother. Sorry, you may not want to hear this but, if you are putting others before your spouse, you are out of order. God speaks to this in Genesis 2:24 (KJV) *"A man shall leave his father and mother and shall cleave unto his wife, and they shall be one flesh."*

Some people do not know how to forgive and move on. If they only hear one version of your story, you will portray yourself as the "saint" and make the other person out to be the enemy. That is not fair on their part. As the old saying goes, *"Two wrongs don't make a right."* What part did you play? The only time you should involve someone in your business is when you are being abused or seeking help to develop tools and skills to create a healthy relationship. If you are being abused, never stay silent! Tell someone! It may save your life.

TWO SHALL BE HAPPY

It is not your responsibility to make your partner happy. However, it is your responsibility to present yourself daily to your mate in a way that contributes to their happiness from the love, respect, trust, and commitment you have

Introduction

towards them as a person. Understand, some people want to see your relationship fail because they are miserable and might have no one to share a happy relationship with. Never take advice from someone who does not have their priorities in order. They will lead you down the wrong path to destruction.

Always stay committed to your relationship. You are probably asking, "why should I be committed?" Well, it helps to create a healthy place where you both will be able to share and open up about your feelings and your thoughts. In a healthy relationship, commitment breeds respect and respect empowers love, and love shows up in appreciation. And appreciation shows your care for both the relationship and your mate.

Every healthy relationship is built on a foundation of respect, love, and trust. Trust does not say that temptation will not arise. Trust says that when temptation arises, I will respect myself, my commitment to my relationship, the love I have for my partner/mate and the respect I have for my partner/mate as I tell the Devil he is a liar.

"Watch and pray so that you will not fall into temptation. The spirit is willing, but the flesh is weak." (Matthew 26:41 KJV)

"Be well balanced and always alert, because your enemy, the devil, roams around incessantly, like a roaring lion looking for its prey to devour. Take a decisive stand against him and resist his every attack with strong, vigorous faith." (1 Peter 5:8-11 TPT)

Let's take the blinders off and get real. There are some people out here who are *only* attracted to married men/women. That ring on your finger is more of a magnet than a deterrence for them. Their flirtations are flattering, and their conversation seems innocent in the beginning. That is until they ask you questions like: Are you happily married? How long have you been married? Where is your spouse? Is he/she the right one for you? Do you know what you are missing out on? All of which are designed to allow doubt or permit previously hurt feelings to enter into your heart/mind. This gives them the opening they need to try to destroy the trust that has been built in your relationship. While having you all caught up in your feelings.

Introduction

It would amaze you at some of the pickup lines we have heard. Both men and women who try to disrupt your marriage do not care about respecting your marriage. They are on the hunt. Preying on any vulnerability they see to get what they want. But when you are committed to building and maintaining a healthy relationship with your husband/wife, they do not stand a chance.

It is baffling that *"relationship intruders"* enjoy being with someone they do not have to be **accountable for or to. They enjoy that there are no "strings" attached. Some people think** that being with someone who is with someone else gives them the sense of being with a more experienced person. They find the person attractive and desirable. They want to be in a relationship that is secretive and undercover. Remember what we discussed earlier about the law of attraction. Think about your relationship with yourself and the conversation you are having with yourself about your committed relationship. Are you leaving breadcrumbs for someone else to find you and be a *"relationship intruder"* in your life? Do not give place to the Devil. Do not allow his followers to use you to boost their self-esteem by convincing you they are the answer to your unhappiness and/or dis-ease. Remember, when you and your spouse are connected, committed, and concerned about each other's best interests, nothing will get in the way.

COMMITMENT

To maintain a healthy relationship, some couples need to recommit themselves to each other. If you have strayed away from the things that brought the two of you together, return to it. If, in the beginning of the relationship, the both of you committed to weekly date nights, cozy cuddle nights, movie nights, and/or just having 'getting to know you' conversations with each other; commit to making time to do those relationship building activities again. By ignoring this advice and not scheduling and/or making time for relationship building activities, couples will begin to feel disconnected. Take the time to rebuild the flame and rebuild the fire you had for each other. Quality time spent together is just as important because it trains both individuals to utilize their communication

Introduction

skills and reminds them why they are in a committed relationship with each other.

As I stressed earlier, trust and respect are the foundation on which your committed relationship stands. They are cornerstones that remind you, during difficult times, why you are committed to your partner/mate. There are no big I's and little u's in relationships! You are equal partners in your relationship. There may come a time when one is giving more than the other because something is going on in the life of the other person. However, that should not be the norm in any relationship. It is imperative that you both remember to always support one another.

There are many other ways to build a healthy relationship: connect with each other regularly, communicate honestly and openly, make it a habit to plan and spend quality time with each other, and make a habit of going out and spending time with friends as a couple and separately. Being under each other 24/7 is unnecessary.

We hope you are ready to dive deeper into this book and learn the Substance of Building Healthy Relationships. Take notes as we share real-life scenarios, and our own personal journeys fret with trials, tribulations, and the joys to help you navigate your committed relationships successfully, respectfully, and lovingly. It is our goal to show you how to fully love yourself and be fully loved by others.

Introduction

Set boundaries, stand your ground, realize who you are, and know your worth.

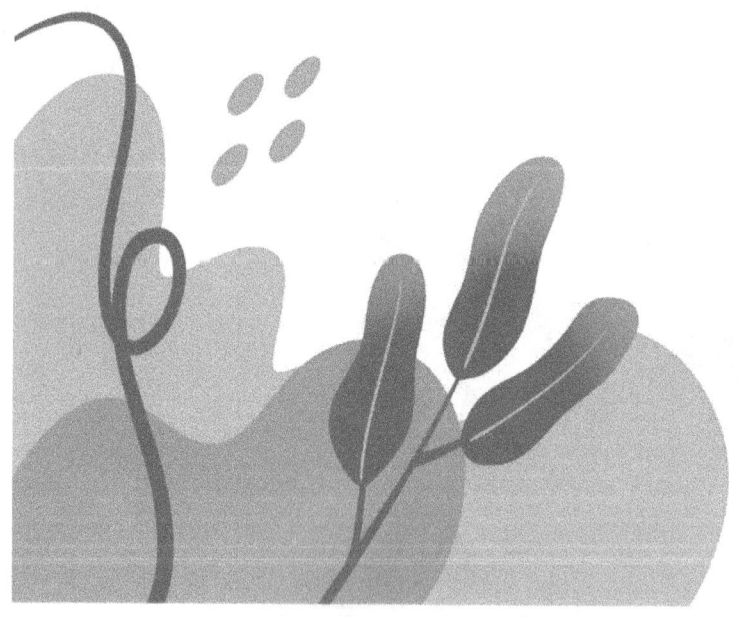

CHAPTER 1

Setting Boundaries

It's me, Darlene.

Let me share with you, my story. I've been married three times. Each one was a rocky road in and of themselves. They were definitely not perfect. I have had two divorces. Trying to rebuild my life afterwards was crushing. Learning to love myself forced me to wake up from my brokenness and face reality.

These marriages have left me beaten, battered, and bruised. I was kicked downstairs, choked, kicked in the face, given some black eyes, experienced swollen lips, knots on my head, and had Clorox bleach thrown in my eyes …my right eye has never been the same. Why? Because I had no boundaries.

Looking back on the devastation I experienced in these marriages; I realize these things wouldn't have happened to me if I had realized my worth and stood my ground. Wow! I realize now that my life was built on a foundation of fear. Hoping things would change, but sadly, it never did. I didn't love myself; I had low self-esteem and was ashamed of the woman who looked back at me in the mirror. Isolation became my safety blanket. Especially when I was hiding the noticeable bruises from my family and friends.

Although my husband and I have our problems, we realize and take responsibility for the part we played and our actions. After a cool down time, we take the time to determine what led up to the argument and our disrespectful actions/behaviors towards each other. Our marriage isn't perfect! No marriage is! Your relationship will never be perfect either, because neither of you is perfect. I bet you are wondering what is the difference in our marriage now? *Prayer*!

There came a time when we learned the importance of setting boundaries, understood what is acceptable and what is not acceptable in our marriage, how to respect one another, and be intentional with our words. Remember, I said we are not perfect. Sometimes we don't agree with each other and that's ok. Today, we are committed to building a healthy relationship. We have gotten past fussing and disrespecting each other. Where we are today has come from maturity, accountability, and a desire to honor each other. I know it is surprising to read, but I can be a pistol and my mouth can be destructive. What I have learned is that I must watch my tongue because it has and can continue to cause a lot of issues in my marriage. I challenge you to be intentional with your words. Make it a habit to speak life and encouragement.

Earlier, I wrote about the abuse I have suffered during my marriages. I stayed because I didn't know any better and because I did not know my worth/value. I do not want the same thing for you! Let me make this perfectly clear!!! I don't care what you said or didn't say; did or didn't do. No one has the right or permission to put their hands on you! Take some advice from someone who has been there and done that. If neither of you are willing nor trying to work it out, then remove yourself from the relationship. My marriage is a testament that if you both are willing to do the work and learn how to listen to each other instead of reacting and hurting each other's feelings; then your marriage has a chance.

No marriage changes overnight. There is work both individuals must put in to ensure you are repairing the foundation of your relationship that will support you both in the days, weeks, months, and years to come. My husband and I have done the work and put the boundaries in place that demands we love, honor, and respect each other. Without those boundaries, I am not sure where our marriage would be today. The boundaries weren't the only thing that needed to change in our relationship. We both had to agree to walk away and not react to whatever was said or done when we were angry. Which has allowed us to turn our marriage around and put it on the right path. The path that helps us align our marriage with the word of God. None of this was easy, but with prayer and us both being committed, we were able to create the relationship we need to grow within our marriage.

Setting Boundaries

Even though we still experience issues within our marriage, each day we work on improving our marriage. There is one important aspect that we do in our marriage that I encourage you to do in yours. Each day, make it a habit to show each other respect, and to show more love toward each other than you did the day before. Building a marriage and/or a committed relationship is not a sprint. It is a marathon. If love is there, your relationship will work out. Love gives you both permission to take the blinders off and see the things you were doing to each other. Love allows you to see where you are wrong and challenges you to discontinue those things that are hurtful to the person you say you love.

Making a marriage and/or a committed relationship work requires both mates to actively work towards building a healthy relationship. If you wake up one day and realize you have given your all to your mate, and there is no change. Or there is no hope for your marriage and/or you are still being mistreated; it is time to go your separate ways. God honors marriage, but He also tells us to love ourselves. No where in the Bible nor in life does love equal or equate to being mistreated. Prayerfully making the decision to leave after you have done everything you know to do to save or revive a dead relationship; means you have finally learned how to love yourself, set boundaries, and know your worth. Walking away isn't giving up. It is loving and respecting yourself enough not to continue to subject yourself to a toxic/unhealthy relationship.

Although my marriage did not start off as a healthy relationship; I still feel I have been blessed to spend my life with my husband. There was a turning point in our marriage where God stepped in and we allowed Him to help us through the storms, challenges, and obstacles we let into the marriage. We are still together because we are now committed to maintaining a healthy relationship that honors God and each other. If I didn't love myself, understand my role in our relationship and realize my worth, my husband and I would not be together today. Proverbs 18:22 (MSG) says, *"When a man finds a wife, he has found a treasure [good thing]! For she is the gift of God to bring him joy and pleasure."* In the same vein, my husband had to learn Proverbs 18:22 and live it. Had he not come to this realization and practice it daily in our marriage, we would not be married today.

Set boundaries, stand your ground, realize who you are, and know your worth.

Boundaries are so important within a marriage/relationship. Without them, you have no control over who you are in the relationship. You find yourself being manipulated and controlled by the other person. Boundaries tell the other person what is acceptable and what is not acceptable for you as it relates to the relationship. It is important that clearly articulate and firmly protect how you will be treated during the relationship.

Having boundaries allows you to freely make decisions/choices for yourself and within the relationship without feeling like every choice you make must be predicated on pleasing the other person. They give you the security and the freedom to speak your mind and stick to what you have said. It is your responsibility to educate your mate on how you will show up in the relationship and your expectations regarding how he/she is to treat you. This approach encourages open communication and respectful treatment of each person in the relationship.

Intimacy

Most people shy away from talking about intimacy. To fully understand how to build and maintain a healthy relationship, we must talk about intimacy. In its simplest form, intimacy can be explained as "into-me-see." It is a person's most vulnerable state. When being intimate with your make, boundaries clearly articulated to inform your partner of your preferences. Your likes and dislikes. I know what you are probably thinking or may be saying, "*...Mrs. Darlene even in your marriage bed?*" Yes, ladies and gentlemen, even in your marriage bed! It may be something your husband might want that you do not want to do or something you want he does not want to do. Why should either of you lie there frustrated and unfulfilled? Not enjoying this intimacy because it is all about the other person's enjoyment and pleasure. Both of you should enjoy and be satisfied during your shared intimate moments. Setting boundaries can help you have a healthy

Setting Boundaries

relationship because you both were upfront at the beginning of the relationship, and even during the relationship you keep it 100 at all-times. Even during those times when you might have to have some uncomfortable conversations because you both are committed to open and honest communication.

The following are some steps that I have found helpful when setting up boundaries to maintain a healthy relationship:

1. Explain what you like and don't like.
2. Speak in a calm voice.
3. Be straight forward.
4. Say no and mean it.
5. Respect other's beliefs and values.
6. Be consistent.
7. Do not argue.

Short Story #1:

Joy met Tony at a picnic given by her cousin. They kicked it off immediately. It wasn't just about the attraction, but the safety they each felt in the other person's presence. Later in the relationship, Joy noticed how Tony would talk to her. After a while, he became very demanding and would get loud when speaking with her. Which caused others to pay attention to him. Joy thought it was something she could handle. So, she would just play it off and ignore what he was doing. Joy also noticed that when Tony drank, he would become a different person. He would overreact and often yell at her. Joy seemed to shrink in Tony's presence. She was afraid to say anything. Let alone speak up for herself. It got so bad that she would not go out in public with him or around the family.

In hindsight, she realized there were grave mistakes she made in the relationship. The few boundaries that were in place were consistently ignored. Tony didn't concern himself with what he was doing and how he was treating her. Joy found herself afraid of Tony and unsure of how to interact with him. Everything she did seemed to bring on his wrath. All she knew was that love wasn't supposed to hurt, but she didn't see a life for herself without him in it. So, she stayed, and she endured the abuse.

I shared that story for two very important reasons: (1) remember you have a voice that deserves to be heard and respected. Joy cannot remember when she stopped speaking up for herself in her relationship with Tony. She only remembers the abuse and when fear became her constant companion; and (2) identify and set boundaries early in your relationship. The way Joy responded, or shall I say, didn't respond to Tony's actions, shows that her boundaries were pushed aside. Which left her feeling like she didn't matter because the first time Tony yelled at her, said to her he did not respect nor regard her boundaries.

I cannot say this enough! It is important to address boundaries early in the relationship. Attempting to set boundaries once a situation gets out of hand and when you are ready to explode is dangerous. If your spouse/mate doesn't know and/or respect your boundaries, they will continue to walk over them and you.

Setting boundaries can help you build and maintain a healthy relationship. It is important that both individuals be mentally and emotionally sound in the marriage/relationship. Earlier, I stated the importance of knowing who you are and loving the person looking back at you in the mirror. This is where that becomes paramount. In any unhealthy relationship, there comes a time when you realize you and your partner do not have the same dreams and goals as you believed you once did. This is when you accept fully that you cannot fix him/her because you are on two totally different levels. I encourage you to pay attention to the direction you both are headed in. Are you going one way, and he/she is going in a different direction?

2 Corinthians 6:14 (KJV) says, *"Be ye not unequally yoked together with unbelievers: for what fellowship hath righteousness with unrighteousness? and what communion hath light with darkness?"* If you are unequally yoked to your mate, your boundaries will always be disregarded and disrespected. Which will damage the relationship. In this regard, I encourage you to ensure that you discuss your spiritual beliefs and

together invite Jesus into your relationship. Remember, a three-fold cord is not easily broken. Especially if you, your mate, and Jesus are the three members of the cord. This can also apply to any relationship you may have. There is always a need to set boundaries to ensure everyone agrees and understands that your boundaries speak to you knowing who you are and the respect that you deserve.

SHORT STORY #2:

Sandra is a Sterile Processing Technician. She has been at her job for a long time, so she knows the importance of having trays ready for surgery. On the weekend, she works a lot of overtime because they are short staffed. Sandra takes pride in her job and always wants to make sure every tray is ready for the morning surgery cases. When picking up extra hours on the weekend, Sandra notices that her co-workers are laid back and not showing the professionalism that she uses daily. The part that really concerns her is that their lead tech is not saying anything to correct their behavior. Sandra decides to only concern herself with her work and continues to set the surgery trays up as she has always done.

One Saturday morning as Sandra was working, a tray was needed for a morning case right away. As Sandra looked around for the completed trays, she realized the supplies were still on the shelf and had not been assembled. Sandra continued working at the pace she had established for herself. She had completed a lot of trays during her shift and had more to work on. As she was working, she noticed the other techs were talking and doing nothing.

The lead tech took the tray that was needed and placed it on Sandra workstation instead of giving it to the other non-working tech and ask her to stop what she was doing and work on the tray that was needed right away. Sandra realizes she was being taken advantage of and her boundaries were being disregarded because she stays over and gets the job done. She believed that because she doesn't complain and focuses on her job; just let her do it. Sandra looked at the lead tech and calmly said not today. Give it to a tech that is not doing anything. She refused to be used to fix a problem that would not have been an issue had everyone been doing their job during their scheduled shift.

In every relationship we have, boundaries need to be set and respected. When boundaries are disrespected and/or disregarded for whatever reason, it creates issues and discord that damages the relationship(s). In Sandra's case, everyone took for granted that she would always do the right thing and not say anything about others not stepping up and doing their job. Simply because she does her job, works the overtime offered and never complains. When setting boundaries at your job, in your home, in your marriage, it creates a healthy environment in which to work, live and/or love.

"…it's not the big things that complicate a relationship. It is the little inconsistencies that build over time."

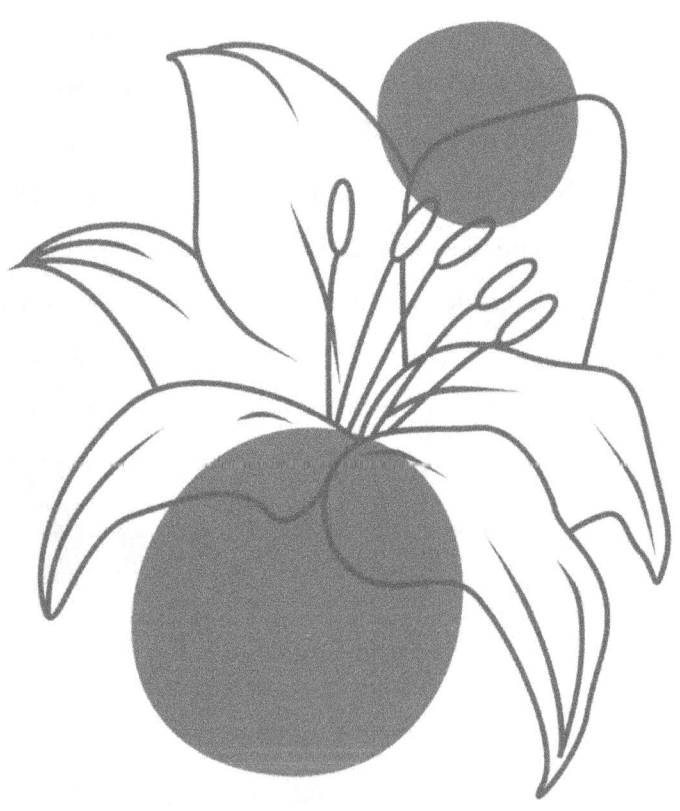

CHAPTER 2

Things Women and Men Need in a Relationship

Women and men need to feel respected, appreciated and loved in their relationships. Without respect, it is impossible to build and/or maintain a healthy relationship. We, as humans, must know that our mate is trustworthy and worthy of the time and energy we invest in them.

Your mate does not have the patience or time to play psychiatrist. Couples need each other to say what they mean and mean what they say. For example, you decide to meet for dinner at 6:00pm and your mate does not show until 7. That is *NOT* acceptable, unless you have an emergency and you notify me of your delay, or the change,

I will forever remember that time you left me waiting on you. Operate from the premise that respect is inherent and requires continued and open communication. Do not let ego impede either of you from showing this level of respect to the other. If you are trying to build a healthy relationship, as a couple, you both need to know your feelings matter to the other person.

Trust is a fragile thing, and it can be broken easily. Remember, the same way you want to be treated by your mate is how you should treat your mate. If you are no longer attracted to them, release them. Because if the truth be told, your attraction lies in or with someone else, and that is where you would rather be. Why allow yourself to be in a marriage or relationship with a spouse or significant other that you are no longer attracted to? Remember, the person who you are in a relationship with has feelings, and when they find out how you really feel, it can be disastrous. If your feelings or the tenor of the relationship has changed for you, share that information with your mate. Don't act like you are looking for a committed relationship when the truth is you are not!

Things Women and Men Need in a Relationship

When in a committed relationship, each partner will pay more attention to what they do than what they say because their actions speak louder than their words. Women and men also need to know their spouse/mate is capable of love. Some men think it is a weakness to express their love and appreciation to their spouse. Showing or expressing love through your emotions is a sign of being human and your willingness to share love with those you are in a relationship with. We all take our chances if we sincerely want to get to know the other person. It makes everything easier when both parties are open to expressing love and affection, which gives your partner a reason to stick around so they can get to know you better. Neither women nor men are looking for a partner to dominate them. They are quite capable of making their own decisions and voicing their own opinions. Everyone deserves someone who will help lift them up and not tear them down.

Sometimes we find ourselves willingly pouring into our partner/mate's cup as much as we hope they will pour into ours. However, that's not always our reality. It is then when we must be honest with ourselves and face the fact that our relationship isn't where we imagined it would be. It's in these moments, I urge you not to blindfold yourself to your reality. Listen to what your heart is whispering. It holds a truth that deserves your attention. Be honest about what is happening and determine what the best course of action is for yourself with a clear and open heart. And by all means, do not make excuses for your mate's bad behavior! It only gives them permission to repeat that behavior and you a ticket to an emotional roller coaster that loops endlessly through highs of hope and lows of letdown.

Never be afraid to set boundaries and standards that honor you and protect your heart in your relationship. It is ok to give, but don't allow yourself to be used or taken advantage of. Remember, you determine your do's, don'ts, and non-negotiables in your relationships. Never allow intimidation to determine any aspect of your relationship. Keeping a positive mindset and an open heart is important. It will let you know when you have had enough, and it is time for you to walk away. Keep your emotions in check and don't allow them to keep you in a relationship longer than you should. As a rule, women tend to love harder than men. A woman's approach to love is to give it freely and wholeheartedly. While men play the field and usually don't put all their eggs in one basket. They believe that by having more than one option is a safety net for them if the relationship doesn't work out. On the other hand, women sometimes take a break in between relationships and don't usually rush into another one quickly.

They regroup and try to figure out why the relationship didn't work so they can avoid taking an unhealed or broken heart into a new relationship. Don't get me wrong; women are not perfect. Women must examine themselves to take responsibility for the part they played in the breakdown or demise of the relationship. To ensure we honor our hearts and heal from the broken relationship, women must be careful and give themselves some grace when figuring out why they acted or reacted the way they did. This level of transparency and honesty will make women own their stuff and forgive themselves for allowing themselves to be treated below their worth. When women do their self-work that leads to a healed heart, they walk away with learned lessons and more love to offer in their next relationship.

Women and men can no longer be naïve to what is being presented to them. Women, our intuition is a very strong and compelling feeling. Don't ignore it. Your intuition is letting you know that something is not right in the relationship. Don't be quick to give the benefit-of-a-doubt. Trust your gut and accept the things you are seeing as true in the relationship. Sometimes you must be uncomfortable to get comfortable by leaving toxic relationships while learning how to not repeat the same cycle of mistrust, disrespect, abuse, etc. in your future relationships.

Unfortunately, some men and women are attracted to the same type of people which can be a disaster; because if you keep choosing the same kind of mate and repeating the same behavior, you are going to continue getting the same results: failed relationships. Believe in yourself, start doing things that make you happy, have some me time and

Things Women and Men Need in A Relationship

enjoy your own company. It is okay to go to dinner alone or go see that movie that your spouse/mate is not interested in seeing. Make yourself the most important person in your life and start living your dreams again. Remember, you deserve better. There's a lot of good men/women out there who desire to treat you respectfully and lovingly. If you have breath in your body, it is not too late. Trust and believe in yourself and in your destiny. You can and will win if you put the work in and close those chapters in your life. And remember, YOU hold the pen to start your next chapter.

No matter how long you've been in that bad relationship, don't be afraid to start over. Fear will keep you from reaching your destiny and experiencing the most amazing things life has to offer. Allow yourself to grow by accepting the fact that you define who you are and don't look for that from anyone else. Become comfortable in your own skin and protect your peace. Do not allow failed toxic relationships to change you! Otherwise, you will protect yourself from the people who will treasure you if given the opportunity to have you in their life.

Regenerate

We, as women and men, must find our own strength; no one can have it for us. For us to move on, we have to learn how to forgive them and ourselves. Whether or not they deserve it. Most of the time, they are not sorry for not being who you need and deserve in your relationship. They only want things to continue being as they were. Sometimes, we want to hurt those who have hurt us by doing to them what they have done to us. Don't sink to their level. Instead, regroup and face the fact that the relationship is no longer valuable to you, release it, learn the lessons it was meant to teach you, and grow.

In some cases, we are let down by the people we trusted the most. Or, should I say, the ones we thought we could trust. Let me say this one more time! If you are giving your all to a relationship and it's still not working, the problem is you are giving it to the wrong person. I give you permission to take your power back. One of the hardest lessons to learn is knowing which hand to hold and which one to let go of when you finally decide to make changes in your life. A part of taking your power back is celebrating your small victories. Those victories that renew your courage and strength. There is no one on earth or in heaven that is better at being you than you. Yes, you made a mistake. You chose the wrong person. So what? Now what?

A confident person doesn't feel the need to prove anything to anyone because they are secure with their life decisions and the mistakes they have made. Whether you win or lose, make the choice yourself. Learn to live with the outcome because it is your life and your decisions. You don't need others to guide your mistakes; trust yourself and realize that you are graced to handle everything that happens in your life. Good or bad! If necessary, seek professional help or talk to someone who has been where you are, but after considering it, make the choice yourself. That way, regardless of the outcome, it's your own decision.

If you repeatedly tell your partner what you want and need from the relationship and they are not fulfilling those needs, it's likely because they do not either have the capacity to do so or they simply do not want to. For instance, if he knows you love flowers, but never brings any home despite your requests, it shows a lack of consideration. However, if he meets another woman, he might bring them flowers on the first date to impress them. This disparity in behavior is telling.

When you notice that his value of you has changed and everyone else's feelings seem more important than yours, gracefully bow out of the relationship. Some of us remain in a relationship out of habit, even when happiness is no longer present. It's astounding how one can get used to a toxic relationship simply because it has been a part of their life for so long, even though deep inside, they know separation should have happened long ago. Sometimes we stay in toxic/unhappy relationships because we fear starting over, getting to know someone new, and trusting again after our trust has been abused.

What was once a good relationship can turn toxic. People change, sometimes they grow apart. Your needs and wants evolve, and you may become unwilling to accommodate your partner's behaviors, needs and/or wants like you did in the past. It takes a lot of work and commitment from both parties to keep a relationship healthy. Open and honest communication is essential in any successful relationship. There should be no need for your spouse to second guess you. If you say you're going to the store, that should be your destination. Often, it's not the big things that complicate a relationship. It is the little inconsistencies that build over time. Poor communication in a relationship can lead to all kinds of problems. When you or your partner no longer feel the need to inform each other of your whereabouts, there's a problem.

Some people believe that committed couples should only socialize with other committed couples and not any single friends. I do think it is better for couples to have friends in committed relationships, so a single friend's lifestyle will not influence them. As I stated earlier, I believe in engaging in separate activities, but sometimes it can add tension to the relationship when there is a hidden agenda. I caution you to never let a friend cause any problems in your relationship with your spouse/mate. You never know, their actions or behaviors may be because they are not happy in their relationship and is trying to sabotage

Substance of Building Healthy Relationships

---

yours. Remember, misery loves company. Each person in a relationship is responsible for their own actions, behaviors, and words. If your mate crosses the line, your issue isn't with anyone else but him/her because you are in a relationship with them, and they are the person who betrayed your trust. If you plan on hanging out with friends, be open about it. Don't think I am saying never take time for yourself. What I am saying is that I encourage it. Just be honest with your spouse/mate about it because honesty builds trust.

In this chapter, we have talked about having open and honest, taking time for yourself, and what a man and woman need in a relationship. I think it is important to consider some reasons a man/woman may decide to leave a relationship. Regardless of how much they have invested in the relationship. Here are some reasons an individual chooses to leave their relationship:

1. Your spouse/mate believes is putting others before you. They are not honoring your role in their life.
2. They cannot trust their mate.

Things Women and Men Need in A Relationship

3. He/She is no longer investing time in their mate or the relationship.
4. There's no spontaneity from your partner. You make all the plans for your vacations, date night, etc.
5. Both are unhappy in the relationship.
6. He/She no longer feels appreciated, wanted, or needed in the relationship.

If you can relate to any or all the statements above and you are still committed to the relationship, get it together or you are going to lose them. No one wants to be with someone who doesn't value them.

"In toxic situations, one might feel silenced; their opinions are disregarded, leading to feelings of insignificance."

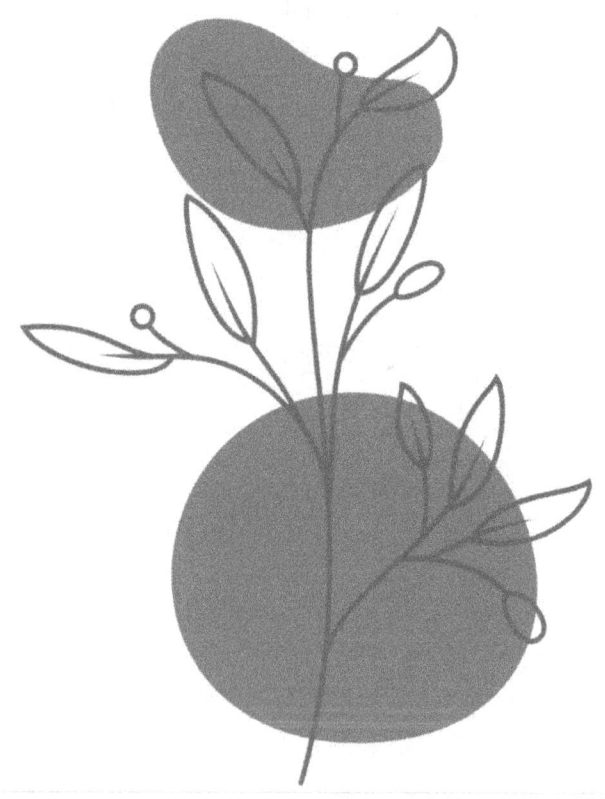

CHAPTER 3

Toxic Verses Healthy

When entering into a new relationship, it is very important to leave past relationships in the past. What you have left and overcome should stay where you left it and gracefully move on. If you haven't overcome it, put on the brakes and work on yourself before you quickly get into another relationship. Free yourself from all the pain and hurt you have endured and begin to love yourself.

TOXIC is something that is poisonous or very harmful or unpleasant in a pervasive or insidious way, according to Dictionary.com. According to VerywellMind.com, a toxic relationship is one that makes you feel unsupported, misunderstood, demeaned, or attacked. A relationship is toxic when your well-being is threatened in some way—emotionally, psychologically, and even physically. It is filled with all kinds of chemicals and fumes that will destroy your self-esteem, self-worth and/or character. It is something you do not want to be part of or participate in. This kind of behavior will cause fear within the relationship because the dominant person is very manipulative and abusive.

In a healthy relationship, each person should feel safe and secure. If this sense of safety is missing, it is an indicator of a toxic environment. Peaceful communication is essential, even when discussing challenging issues. While disagreements are normal, since not everything will be agreeable, it becomes problematic when one partner consistently insists; they are always right and refuse to consider the other's viewpoint. If they become loud, dominating, and dismissive of your thoughts, it is a clear sign of toxicity.

In toxic situations, one might feel silenced; their opinions are disregarded, leading to feelings of insignificance. Initially, relationships often start positively. As they progress and emotions deepen, some individuals may reveal their true selves. It is not uncommon to question the abrupt change in behavior and wonder if it's your fault or if you can fix it. It is important to understand that it is not your fault. The signs were perhaps there from the beginning, but love can sometimes cloud judgment.

Love can lead to acceptance of behaviors that are detrimental to one's well-being. It is easy to be blinded by love and miss the following signs of a toxic relationship, which can include:

1. Low self-esteem.
2. Avoidance of the partner.
3. Constant anxiety and uncertainty in conversations.
4. Public embarrassment.
5. Feelings of anger and depression.
6. Inability to be yourself around them.
7. Efforts to please them, just to maintain peace.
8. Blaming yourself for everything.
9. Acceptance of their lies.
10. Experiencing disrespect.

11. Dealing with a self-centered partner.
12. Encountering jealousy and insecurity.

Acknowledging these red flags and/or warning signs is crucial when evaluating the health of your relationship. And when determining if you need to walk away from the relationship. Don't miss this next point. Toxic relationships are not only found in marriages and/or committed relationships. It can also be the foundation on which dysfunctional relationships with family members, friends, and/or co-workers stand.

Being in a toxic relationship can significantly affect a person's self-esteem, mental and physical health. Reminding yourself daily to put on your 'happy face' mask that you believe is making people see and believe you are happy. All while you are crumbling on the inside, longing for a way out but feeling uncertain about how to safely make it happen. This often leads to a deeper state of depression and social isolation.

In the hope of fixing the relationship, you make compromises that negatively affect your health and mindset. Love is sometimes blind. Love should never be associated with being overbearing, overwhelming and/or pushing someone over the proverbial emotional edge. In an intimate relationship, you have entrusted your deepest secrets and personal stories to this person, believing they will always support you and have your back. Unfortunately, they turn out to be the very person who hurts you the most, making you feel worthless. In the beginning, you believed them to be your "prince charming" or "perfect mate." Only to realize you are in a toxic relationship.

As women, the desire for love and affection can sometimes cause us to jump into a relationship without really knowing the person. Declaring in sometimes less than two weeks that you are in love. My mother used to say, "*Everything that looks good isn't necessarily good for you. Choose wisely.*" Pay attention to how they behave, what they say, and how they treat you in public and/or around family and friends.

The red flags and/or warning signs have always been there, but you could not see them because of your lack of emotional intelligence: making decisions from a place of loneliness, depression and/or not wanting to be alone. Despite seeing the warning signs, many still attempt to try to change the other person; while failing to realize that true love cannot flourish in a toxic environment.

If you find yourself in a toxic relationship and it is causing you a lot of stress, there are ways to overcome this and find peace. Understand and accept that you are not in a healthy relationship. Do an internal and honest self-check and remove that cracked 'happy face' mask to see your relationship for what it is and not what you want it to be. Do not blame yourself for their behavior. Speak up for yourself and let them know their behavior toward you is unacceptable, and you will not continue to tolerate their disrespect in public, private, or around family and friends. If they continue to treat you this way, leave the relationship.

A relationship should be founded on love and respect. Love is not abusive. Love should not have you stressed out and in tears.

SHORT STORY

Melissa had been divorced for eight years, her marriage ending because of domestic violence. With a child she adored, she was cautious about introducing a male figure into their lives. Fearful of being let down again, she isolated herself from dating and struggled to trust anyone, especially men. Despite her family's encouragement to move on, Melisa could not shake the trauma of her past relationship.

Her ex-husband had been abusive and controlling, isolating her from loved ones and constantly criticizing and belittling her, even in front of her child. Despite her love for him, Melisa endured years of abuse, hiding her bruises, and making excuses for her absence at family gatherings. His threats kept her in constant fear.

The turning point came when her husband pushed her down the stairs, resulting in her hospitalization. The hospital alerted the police and her family. Initially, Melisa denied the abuse, but after her family's intervention, she realized she deserved better, especially for her child's sake.

After being discharged, Melisa filed charges against her husband with her family's support. He was arrested, and despite his pleas for forgiveness, Melisa stood firm. She relocated with her son, leaving no trace for her ex-husband. Five years later, Melisa opened her heart again and remarried, finding happiness with a man who treated her like a queen. Melisa's story ends on a positive note, but not everyone is so fortunate. Statistics from the Bureau of Justice show that daily, more than three women and one man lose their lives by the actions of their intimate partners.

Many women are trapped in similar situations, unsure of where to turn. It is important to remember that there is hope and help available. As a survivor of domestic violence, I understand the feelings of low self-esteem, shame, and desperation. Counseling and powerful words of encouragement helped me reclaim my life. I would remind myself daily that "*I am a sparkle in God's eyes. He loves and wants the best for me. Love is not abuse. I am in control of my life*." Saying these words to myself daily saved my life and reminded me I deserve better.

To those in toxic relationships: recognize the signs, stand your ground, and embrace self-love. Remember, love is healthy, not toxic. You deserve love and respect.

DOMESTIC VIOLENCE

Being in a relationship characterized as domestic violence is detrimental. Often referred to as intimate partner violence, domestic violence manifests in multiple ways, including physical, sexual, emotional, verbal, and psychological abuse. While commonly associated with women, men can also be victims.

Regardless of gender or sexual orientation, domestic violence can surface in any relationship, whether married, dating, or cohabiting. It often begins with threats and verbal assault, escalating to physical violence. Survivors face emotional and psychological stress, with severe instances leading to issues like depression and anxiety.

Emotional abuse, in particular, can erode a person's self-esteem and self-worth.

If you find yourself in such a relationship, it is critical that you recognize the signs and break free. Do not be swayed by their promises to change; abusers often revert to their old ways after a while. A healthy relationship should not involve fear, belittlement, or control. Ask yourself: Are you constantly afraid? Do you feel trapped, thinking everything is your fault? Does your partner belittle you, use you as a scapegoat for their behavior/actions, or isolate you from friends and loved ones? Are there continuous threats of harm, either to you, your children, or themselves? Are you forced to deal with their incessant jealousy, them withholding finances, and/or their constant surveillance, or need to know your every move? If you answered yes to all or most of the questions, you are in an abusive relationship.

Remember, you deserve respect, love, and kindness. Do not settle for anything less. Love does not entail threats or belittlement. Do not sentence yourself to a lifetime of this treatment for fear of being alone. Being alone and loneliness are two different things. If the only choices, you have is to be in an abusive relationship or be alone. Then choose to be alone, because solitude is preferable to abuse. There are individuals who will value and love you genuinely. Prioritize your well-being and free yourself from the chains of domestic violence. Embrace your worth, wear your crown with pride, and foster self-love.

"While we all crave love, remember that not everyone is capable of giving it."

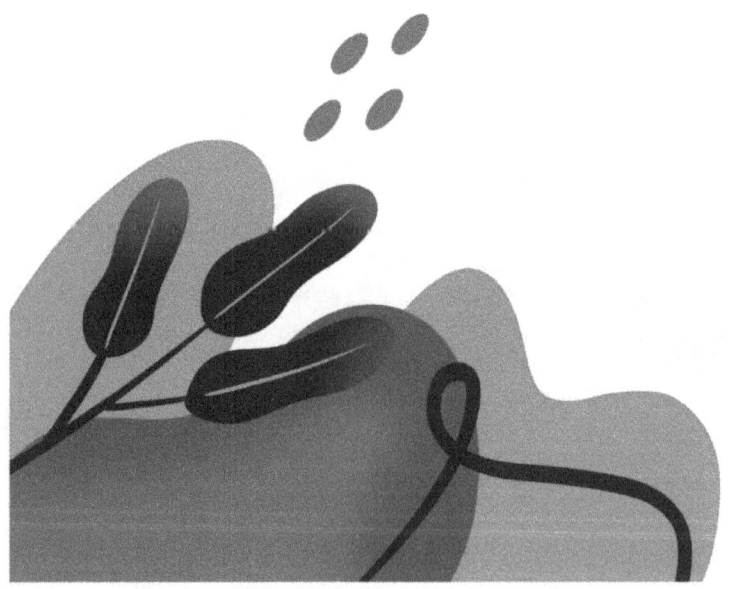

CHAPTER 4

Importance Of Self-esteem

While researching what self-esteem is, I learned: Self-esteem is a person's overall sense of their value or worth. It is similar to self-respect and describes a person's level of confidence in their abilities and attributes. Self-esteem is also based on a person's opinions and beliefs about themselves, which can sometimes feel difficult to change. Two categories: low and high characterize self-esteem. People with low self-esteem are filled with doubts and criticisms about themselves and their abilities. They believe they are inadequate and less worthy than others. People with high self-esteem think well of themselves and their abilities. They believe they are good and worthy, and that others view them positively. Therefore, high self-esteem is pivotal for a happy and fulfilling life. Unfortunately, we often let others treat us as we treat ourselves, despite our flaws. Remember, you are beautiful, and no one is perfect. Each morning, look in the mirror and affirm, "I love me. I am perfectly made." Embrace your inner strength and start making the changes you desire to boost your self-esteem. Positive self-talk can propel you towards achieving your dreams, living your best life, and finding inner peace. It encourages you to discard chaos and avoid anything that disrupts your tranquility.

I, Barbara, have learned that peace must come from within. While I cannot control everything, I refuse to let others dictate how I feel about myself. My life has been wrought with heartbreaks and pain, and love, beauty, and new beginnings, which I wholeheartedly embrace. These experiences have shaped me into the beautiful woman I am today.

When you give someone else the power to dictate your happiness, you lose your sense of self. But when you build your self-esteem, you realize you have always had the power. This realization marks the beginning of not settling

IMPORTANCE OF SELF-ESTEEM

for less or underestimating your worth. Women, we are often our own worst critics, and we need to learn how to acknowledge our strengths and cultivate self-love. It takes courage to leave behind what does not serve you, but the courage to change leads you towards a better life.

Abusers seldom participate in introspection; they prefer to blame others. Often, we hurt ourselves by overvaluing our significance or importance in their lives. The way someone treats you reflects their feelings towards you. Whether their behavior strengthens or diminishes your self-esteem is up to you. A controller or abuser can only control/abuse you as long as YOU allow it to happen. When you stop accepting the treatment, their power diminishes.

There are times when self-confidence is mistakenly perceived as arrogance. Yet, it may be a sign of someone overcoming low self-esteem and embracing growth. Life isn't always smooth; it has its ups and downs. But remain focused and resilient through heartbreaks and disappointments. Do not give up. Instead, give yourself at least 30 minutes daily to reflect on your qualities.

Meditation and achieving goals you have set can significantly boost your self-esteem.

Don't base your worth on another person's opinions. Rise above negativity and recognize your value, even if others do not. Some people might prefer seeing you with low self-esteem, misinterpreting it as weakness or vulnerability. But remember, you dictate the terms and how far you will go on your journey to self-fulfillment and growth. Finding inner peace changes a person's perspective. It gives them permission to control their thoughts and destiny.

There is an analogy that I think is important to share here. It begins with this question, "Why is the rear-view mirror smaller than the windshield?" The windshield is larger than the rearview mirror because it's important to have a clear view of where you are going while offering the most optimal surveillance of what's in front of you. The rearview mirror is smaller so you can see what's behind you, avoid negative situations that are trying to creep back toward you, and learn from it. The same is true in life. Keep past relationships in your past and focus on what is

Importance of Self-Esteem

before you. The only time the two should meet is when you are being reminded that you have already been there and done that and you do not want to go there again. Look back only to appreciate your progress and the obstacles you've overcome. Keep your guard up to protect yourself from hurt and disrespect. Understand your worth and refuse to let anyone make you feel unworthy. Sometimes, disrespect is the closure you need.

Encourage yourself to be strong-minded. While we all crave love, remember that not everyone is capable of giving it. Toxic individuals often reflect their self-treatment onto others. Be selective and know that you're attractive and ambitious. The right person will come along; don't rush. Use this time to set boundaries for future relationships.

High self-esteem deters toxic individuals looking to manipulate and control. Avoid self-inflicted wounds by not ignoring red flags. Choose wisely, look beyond mere attractiveness to see their character and other qualities:

1. Is he/she hardworking?
2. Does he/she have a good personality?

3. Is he/she able to provide for themselves?
4. Does he/she give you their undivided attention on dates?
5. Is he a gentleman/respectful?
6. Is he/she adventurous?
7. Does he/she respect you?

They say a word to the wise is sufficient. Never make anyone a priority in your life when you are an option in theirs. Wait for the prize, and choose a partner based not just on looks, but on their character, values, and attributes.

If you are seeking a partner, it is essential to look beyond mere physical attraction. My mother often said, "*What looks good to you may not be good for you.*" Indeed, connecting with a person's emotions and understanding their reactions to various situations is crucial. Do not hesitate to ask questions; it is better to discover truths early than to face surprises in a committed relationship.

A supportive partner consistently reminds you of your worth to him and the world. This reassurance, conveyed through both words and actions, fosters a nurturing environment. However, some individuals cannot recognize the significant impact their attitudes have on their family and friends. Bringing negativity home from work, for instance, can create stress and discomfort for everyone involved. It is important you leave work-related issues at the office and focus on bringing peace and joy into the home.

Remember, women were created from the emotion (love) God has for man (Adam). As such, women are more emotionally attuned and may need more support and understanding than their male counterparts. Conversely, men also benefit from positive, supportive relationships. It is crucial to match positivity with positivity and to distance oneself from those who undermine self-worth. Accepting poor treatment from your mate can lead to self-doubt and diminished self-esteem. Remember, you cannot force anyone to treat you with respect, but you always have the choice to walk away and seek peace of mind rather than settling for a fraction of what you deserve. Sometimes, distance can bring clarity, and a person may come to realize the value of what they have lost because of ignorance or misplaced loyalties once you are gone.

From personal experience, I have learned that mature men appreciate women with healthy self-esteem. Men who lack confidence may attempt to diminish a woman's self-worth. Often, it takes time for someone to realize they are in an unhealthy relationship. It may show up after he/she has realized that their needs are consistently being neglected, and they systematically begin to gradually close the door to their heart. Once closed, the love he/she once had might be irretrievable because they finally see what is happening in their relationship. Before it is too late, I implore you to focus on nurturing your relationship and keep the channels of love open.

Once the individual walks away from the toxic/unhealthy relationship, experiences the relief of not constantly walking on eggshells, and is free from toxicity, a person's self-esteem flourishes. They feel empowered, focused, and unwilling to lower their standards. This breakthrough often comes from living by higher standards and embracing independence. Independence and self-reliance

IMPORTANCE OF SELF-ESTEEM

are crucial. I learned early on not to follow the crowd. It is essential to forge your path, even if it means walking alone. Do not let others sway you to change your direction; stay true to your goals and beliefs. A strong sense of self improves a person's self-esteem and helps them resist the pull of destructive influences.

While it is important to be empathetic, prioritize your well-being and happiness. Past mistakes should not dictate future decisions. In relationships, integrity is paramount. Dishonesty and deception are signs of a lack of integrity. Stand firm in your values and don't compromise your happiness. Remember, growth and progress often involve letting go. Surround yourself with positive, ambitious individuals who uplift your spirit. Maintain a good attitude and be grateful for what you have, as this mindset paves the way for advancement. Despite life's challenges, choose not to dwell on past hardships, but instead focus on your happiness and a brighter future. Do not get discouraged by temporary setbacks. Your breakthrough is closer than you think, and blessings are on their way. Maintain faith and courage as you approach victory.

Finally, it is important to share your experiences and insights with future generations. Teach them about the importance of self-esteem, the value of using their voice, and the need to stand firm in relationships. Words are powerful tools—use them wisely.

Importance of Self-Esteem

"No marriage is perfect, obstacles will occur, how you handle them is the key."

CHAPTER 5

Overcoming All Obstacles

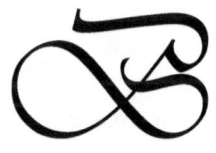eing in a relationship can present numerous challenges, including communication breakdowns, financial stress, insufficient quality time, and a lack of intimacy. These issues can potentially lead to divorce or separation. One of the key reasons relationships fail is a lack of trust. Without trust, partners may grow apart, eventually falling out of love.

It's essential when entering a relationship to ensure mutual understanding of each other's goals. Commitment levels may vary; your partner might have a different perspective on the relationship than you do. If one feels pain, hurt, rejection, or neglect, it can lead to feelings of loneliness and a sense of being unloved. This struggle for attention

Substance of Building Healthy Relationships

can lead to a difference of opinion and thoughts that no one cares.

When facing obstacles in your relationship, reflect on its healthiness. Ask yourself if you made the right decision entering this relationship. Consider if there were warning signs you overlooked, or if you were so enamored that you ignored your partner/mate's flaws. Understanding and accepting that neither you nor your partner/mate is perfect is crucial.

If you encounter many obstacles in your marriage or relationship down the road, do not lose hope. Recovery is possible. There are ways to address and resolve the issues you and your partner/mate are facing.

COMMUNICATION

Having open communication is a cornerstone of a healthy relationship. It's important to discuss various aspects of your lives, including successes and failures. Both partners should feel comfortable talking to each other, knowing that they may hold different opinions. Disagreements are inevitable, but it's crucial not to judge each other based on these differences. Listening is just as important as sharing your own views and understanding that communication is a two-way street.

Remember that all relationships have their highs and lows, and conflicts will arise. However, the ability to communicate openly with your partner can significantly improve your relationship. Do not suppress your feelings; instead, express what's bothering you and what you find unacceptable.

When your partner speaks, listen attentively, without judgment, and be fully present. When disagreements occur, acknowledge their feelings, and accept that their perspective may differ from yours. Understanding and respecting each other's viewpoints is key to a healthy relationship.

TRUST

Trust is the foundation of a healthy relationship. It is vital to feel confident that your partner has your best interests at heart and is reliable. Doubts should not cloud your mind about each other. Both partners should feel free to come and go, but respect each other enough to inform their spouse/mate about their whereabouts. Leaving without any communication can create mistrust.

Setting boundaries early in the relationship is crucial. Discuss what is acceptable and what isn't. Never settle for less. One of the worst feelings in a relationship is the lack of trust, which leads to panic every time your partner/mate leaves. A solid relationship is built on mutual trust and understanding, not on fear and suspicion.

QUALITY TIME

In the early stages of a relationship, going out and spending time together is a frequent and exciting activity. However, as time passes, this can often slow down. It is not uncommon for individuals to think, "*I have him/her, so these things don't matter anymore.*" One may get caught up in their own activities, leading to a decline in quality time spent together. Yet, in any relationship, quality time is crucial. It helps relationships grow stronger and deeper. Despite life's busy schedule and endless errands, nothing should take precedence over spending quality time with your significant other.

Quality time is essential for couples, as it expresses affection and love. It's about giving your partner/mate's attention, making them feel loved and appreciated. In today's world, technology can be a significant distraction. It's all too common to have a phone or tablet in hand, even during conversations. When with your partner, it's important to put away the phone and focus on them. Show them they are more important than any device. Maintain eye contact and show that everything else can wait.

Despite busy lives, it's important to carve out quality time together. Planning is key. Aim for at least one date night a week. Avoid monotony by varying activities. Try new restaurants, visit different movie theaters, take walks while holding hands, or even work out together. The possibilities are endless. Even mundane activities like grocery shopping can be an opportunity for connection and can bring a smile to your partner/mate's face.

Always be present and available to each other. Remember, tomorrow is not promised. Cherish and maximize the time you have together.

SEX

In the beginning, sex often occurs frequently in relationships, sometimes even daily. Over time, you may notice changes; perhaps the frequency has decreased or stopped altogether. It's essential to ask yourself: Is the desire still there? Are you still attracted to your partner? Sex is meant to be a connection point designed to keep the flame alive in a relationship. If you're experiencing problems in this area, consider what might have changed and what you can do to rekindle your sexual connection.

Overcoming All Obstacles

Here are some tips to light the flames:

1. Hug and kiss your partner daily.
2. Surprise each other with unexpected gifts.
3. Set the mood with candles and a bubble bath.
4. Take showers together.
5. Give each other body rubs.
6. Go to bed feeling attractive. (Take the bonnet off. lol)
7. Touch each other softly.
8. Try something new.
9. Communicate your wants and desires.
10. Engage in role-play.
11. Explore sex toys.
12. Share what works and what doesn't.
13. Don't fake it.
14. Cuddle after sex.
15. Create a romantic atmosphere.
16. Discuss any health concerns that may affect your sex life.

Remember, safe sex is crucial. Your body is a temple, not to be taken for granted. My mother, Leah Early, used to say, "*If he can lie down with you, he can marry you.*"

Building a healthy relationship requires work, patience, and commitment. No relationship is perfect, but you can work together to improve it. When challenges arise, don't be selfish; consider your partner's feelings and opinions. In my marriage, I have learned the importance of compromise and listening. Sometimes, staying quiet doesn't solve problems. It is crucial to express yourself and find common ground.

Empathy is also vital. If you find yourself in a heated situation, take a break to cool down. Avoid arguing over trivial matters. Also, never compare your relationship with others. What you see on social media isn't always the whole story.

What I've learned is to keep private matters off social media. Share positive things instead. If you need to talk, find someone trustworthy. Remember, every couple faces obstacles, but with communication and empathy, you can overcome them together.

"Understanding your worth and demanding respect and love is crucial in any relationship. Remember, people will treat you the way you allow them to."

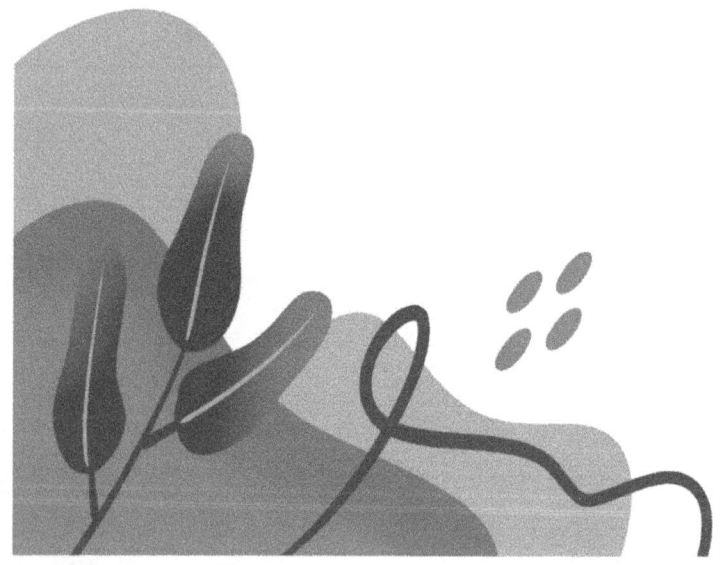

CHAPTER 6

Knowing Your Position

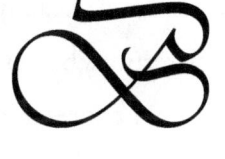eing in a marriage or relationship inevitably brings its share of ups and downs. However, it is crucial to remember that tough times do not last forever.

God created men and women with distinct qualities. Men typically embody strength and resilience, while women often bring gentleness and empathy. Despite their differences, both seek love and respect. In a relationship, understanding and valuing these differences is key to harmony.

Traditionally, men have been seen as the providers and protectors of the family, while women were often the caregivers and homemakers. However, these roles have evolved. Nowadays, women are increasingly taking on roles traditionally held by men, proving their resilience and ability to handle challenging situations. This is not to belittle men; many excel in their roles as providers and caregivers. However, sometimes both men and women fall short of these expectations.

Understanding your worth and demanding respect and love is crucial in any relationship. Remember, people will treat you the way you allow them to. In a healthy partnership, both individuals should share responsibilities. If both partners are working, then household chores and other duties should be divided fairly. Cooperation and teamwork can ease the burden on both parties.

When it comes to finances, communication and transparency are essential. Whether you're dating or married, sharing the financial load, or deciding who pays for what should be a mutual decision. In a relationship, beware of constantly footing the bill, as this could be a sign of being taken advantage of.

In marriage or a long-term relationship, it is advisable to work together on finances. However, if you are not married, it is wise to maintain financial independence to avoid complications if the relationship does not work out.

The foundation of any strong relationship or marriage is friendship. Being friends means you can talk openly, share secrets without fear of judgment, and support each other through thick and thin. Always listen actively, communicate with kindness, and respect each other's opinions, even when you disagree.

Remember, it is not always about being right or having things your way; it is about understanding and respecting each other's perspectives. By recognizing and valuing each other's roles in the relationship, you set the stage for a healthy and balanced partnership.

"When you prioritize your own well-being, external opinions cease to overshadow your joy and energy."

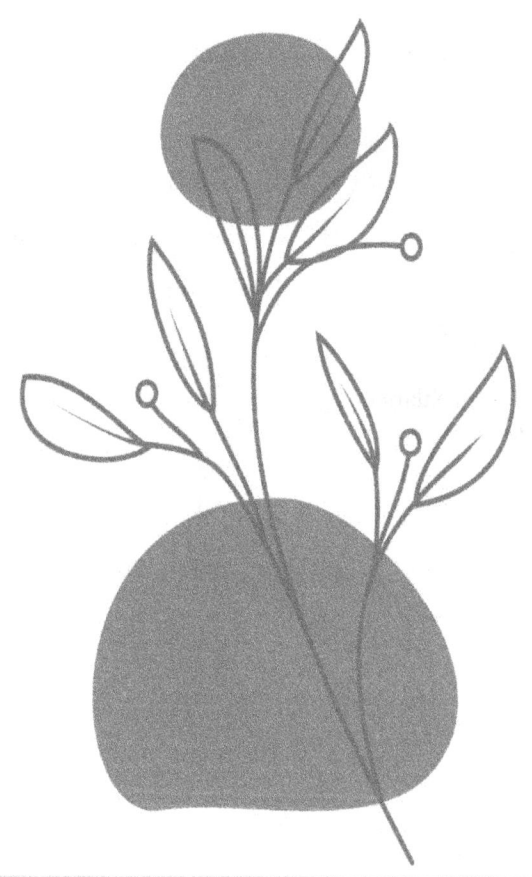

CHAPTER 7

Accomplishments And Goals

In life, we sometimes need to distance ourselves from certain people, places, and things to achieve our goals. Not everyone is meant to stay in our lives. The key to progression is self-acceptance and the willingness to change what no longer aligns with our destinations when reaching our goals, finding inner peace, and cultivating a positive mindset. Replace negative thoughts with ambitious ones, and remember to embrace the hurdles you overcome along the journey.

Recognize what is wrong in your relationship. If you are with the wrong person, even your best efforts may not suffice, as they may not truly love or appreciate you. Conversely, the right partner will value you even at your worst. Do not stay in a toxic relationship, hoping to change the person. People change only if they want to. If it is meant to be, your absence might trigger a change.

Failed relationships often stem from:

1. Conflict and arguments
2. Financial problems
3. Substance abuse
4. Domestic violence
5. Poor communication

67.5% of marriages end because of communication issues. Communication is vital for a strong bond and connection. Impaired communication can lead to arguments, resentment, and hostility. If you constantly argue or avoiding communication to prevent conflict, recognize the problem. If the relationship is valuable, find better ways to communicate. Otherwise, walk away with pride and dignity. It takes two committed people to make a relationship work. If efforts to save it fail, move on for your own well-being.

Signs of a bad relationship include feeling nothing for your partner, lack of communication, feeling alone, distrust, disappointment, and feeling trapped. If these resonate, remember your worth. Free yourself to find someone who truly values you.

To avoid repeating the same mistakes, love yourself. Make yourself happy, knowing happiness lies within you, not solely in your spouse/mate. In transforming, not everyone will be happy, but do not lose yourself trying to please others. Run from red flags in toxic relationships. Reprogram your mind towards excellence. You are meant to have a great life, so let go of bitterness and embrace your potential.

ACCOMPLISHMENTS AND GOALS

Embracing self-love transforms how you perceive negativity and criticism. When you prioritize your own well-being, external opinions cease to overshadow your joy and energy. It is a shift from vulnerability to self-assurance, from seeking external validation to appreciating your own worth.

Growth happens when an individual reaches this level of self-acceptance. You no longer feel diminished by others' negative behaviors; instead, you greet criticism with a smile, recognizing your inner beauty and ambition. Self-prioritization becomes your focus and empowers you to validate your own importance instead of waiting for someone else to validate you.

Self-compliments and solitude teach you to find contentment from within, independent of external affirmation. Loving yourself cultivates an unwavering happiness, a sense of empowerment to face challenges confidently.

The journey to self-love varies for everyone. Here are some steps to consider:

1. Embrace positivity over negativity.
2. Accept your imperfections while recognizing your unique creation.
3. Distance yourself from toxic people and situations.
4. Invest quality time in activities that bring you joy.

Accomplishments and Goals

5. Prioritize your needs over others'.
6. Remove limitations on your ability to enjoy life and be happy.

Loving yourself illuminates your life and shines from within. It brings a transition from hiding in others' shadows to confidently stepping into the light, expressing and embracing your true self. You learn to accept others without letting them impact you negatively. Judgments lose their sting; you recognize your worth and resilience.

Neglecting self-love can lead to dissatisfaction, depression, and a feeling of inadequacy. This can manifest in various ways:

1. Weight gain or loss.
2. Low self-esteem and self-worth.
3. Feelings of failure.
4. Abandoning dreams.
5. Staying in unhealthy relationships.
6. Overwhelming stress.

Not all stress is detrimental; some can be positive, such as:

1. Buying a new home.

2. Job promotions or new opportunities.
3. Welcoming new family members.
4. Getting married.
5. Going on vacations.
6. Celebrating holidays.
7. Pursuing hobbies or enhancing skills.
8. Career changes or realizing dreams.
9. Starting new relationships.

Happiness is a precious state, and it's noticeable to those around you, especially children. They sense when something is amiss, even if we try to conceal it. I, Barbara, experienced this when I was in a difficult phase. I internalized my struggles, as I have always been private. With the loss of my closest confidants, I felt alone and became self-destructive. However, I realized that change had to come from within. Through strength and self-reflection, I achieved my dream of becoming a published author, but my journey does not end there.

Detaching from toxic relationships and behaviors is crucial. Refuse to accept insincere affection, regardless of

Accomplishments and Goals

its source. Focus on your own betterment, without seeking approval or comparing yourself to others.

Financial independence is another aspect of self-love, but it is essential to remain humble and avoid arrogance. Wealth does not necessarily equate to happiness. Instead, learn from other people's successes without envy. As you heal and grow, be vigilant against falling back into negative mental traps.

To break toxic cycles, sometimes solitude is necessary. Do not let fear hinder you. Trust in your abilities and God's plan. Consistency and faith will elevate you to new heights. Help others, but do not forget to invest in your dreams. Avoid feeling discouraged if the same support is not reciprocated; see it as another opportunity for growth.

In conclusion, prioritize yourself, make thoughtful decisions, and stay focused and ambitious. Set high goals and diligently work to achieve them. I wish you nothing but an abundance of blessings on your journey to developing and maintaining healthy relationships and self-discovery.

"Between relationships, career, and parenting, balance it out to where it benefits everyone."

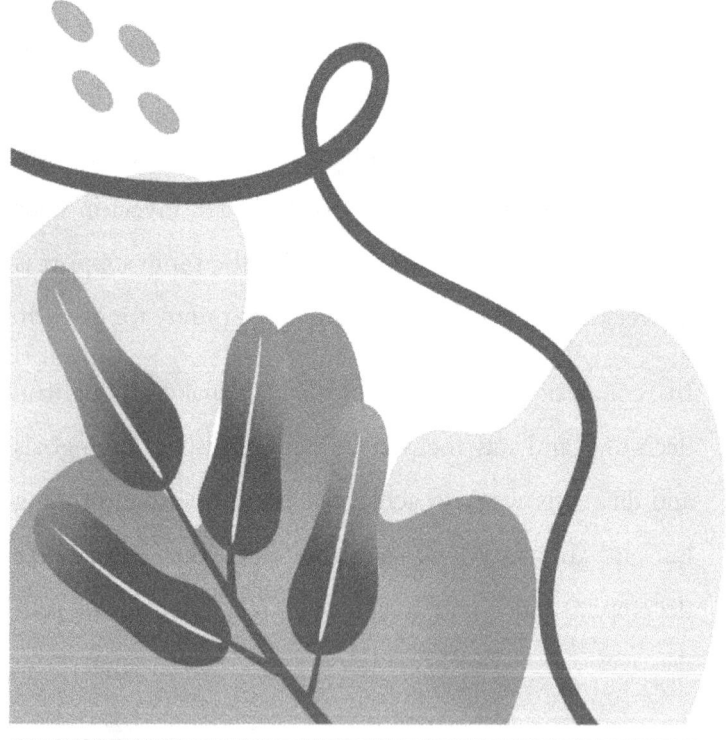

CHAPTER 8

Navigating A Relationship/Career/Parenting

Balancing a relationship, career, and parenting is no easy feat. Each demands quality time, which can either strengthen a relationship or cause it to falter. The arrival of a child changes everything; you are not just partners anymore, your parents. The time once dedicated to each other is now divided between work and caring for your children, leaving many wondering how to maintain a healthy balance.

The responsibility of children means it is no longer just you and your partner. Your attention shifts to caring for another person. The decision to become a parent comes with many considerations: Are you ready for the responsibility? Can you balance a busy schedule with a healthy relationship? Should you stay home with the children or return to work? Who will care for them? These questions are common among new parents.

Financial considerations come into play as well. Raising children can be expensive, and often both parents need to work to make ends meet. For single mothers, the challenge is even greater. They must provide for their children, often without support, and make sacrifices to balance their career and parenting. In contrast, there are fathers who successfully raise their children alone, deserving equal respect and recognition.

For those who are lucky, grandparents can be a blessing in childcare. My own children, Tyiasha, Tommie, and Jennifer, were fortunate to have their grandparents nearby. However, not everyone has that support. I remember the fear and uncertainty when my youngest, Darrius, was injured at daycare. I had to balance my career with ensuring his safety, eventually enrolling him in the daycare where I worked.

Navigating a Relationship/Career/Parenting

Remember, a career is important, but it's not the source of happiness when it comes to family. Family always comes first. At work, give your best, but when you are home, be present for your family. Ensure the safety and wellbeing of your child, whether it is with family members or daycare. If there is any sign of trouble, do not hesitate to take action. If both parents are involved, coordinate childcare and maintain a good relationship for the sake of your child. This cooperation can reduce stress and help you be more productive at work.

Now, let's focus on the relationship aspect. The introduction of a child can strain a relationship because of the shared attention. It is essential to maintain the relationship even when other obligations seem overwhelming. Prioritize your schedule for each other, despite being tired from work. Show appreciation and affection, and never stop showing love and support. Good communication, shared responsibilities, and mutual support are key in balancing career and marriage.

Discuss your career goals, plans for children, and ensure you are on the same page before marriage. If you are not equally yoked, it is a recipe for discord.

In summary, balancing a relationship, career, and parenting is challenging, but not impossible. Prioritize your family, ensure the safety of your children, maintain open communication with your partner, and support each other. Remember, family first, everything else follows.

Navigating a Relationship/Career/Parenting

"These experiences and more have helped me become a better person once I started utilizing the tools and skills I learned, accepted and understood who I am, and regained my self-worth."

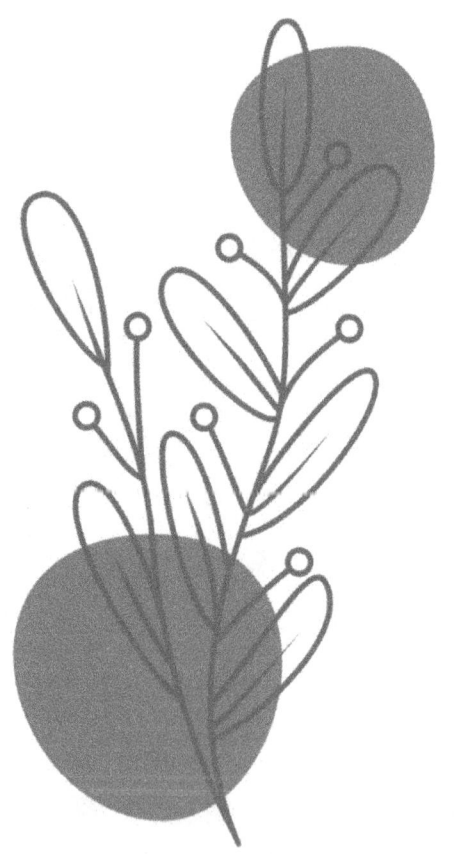

CHAPTER 9

How to Become a Better Person in the Relationship

To become a better version of yourself, it is crucial to embark on a journey of self-discovery. Reevaluate your life and relearn what triggers your emotions—happiness, sadness, or anger. Reflect on your past mistakes, whether in relationships, work, or family, and strive not to repeat them. Recognizing a mistake is the first step; not repeating it prevents it from becoming a lifestyle choice.

Be mindful of the company you keep. Not everyone who smiles at you has your best interest at heart. It is essential to be selective about who you let into your personal space. Remember, you are not perfect either; acknowledging and working on your toxic traits is part of becoming a better person.

I have reached a point in my life where peace is paramount. This realization came after losing my way because of various setbacks, including failed relationships and poor decisions. I had to reconnect with myself to rediscover my worth and purpose. Overcoming the victim mentality was a turning point. I no longer wanted to be defined by my circumstances. Despite feeling beyond repair at times, I have learned the importance of healing and moving forward.

Here's my advice: find a way to heal. Do not linger in a bad place too long, as I did. Time passes quickly, and you do not want to look back with regret. Learn from your mistakes, but do not let them define you. We often carry not just our burdens, but those of our loved ones. However, it is important to realize that we cannot fix everything. Show empathy and understanding, but do not shoulder burdens that are not yours.

How To Become A Better Person In The Relationship

Everyone has unique strengths and weaknesses. Do not compare yourself to others; find what works for you. Remember, your purpose in life is distinct, and not everyone is meant to be a doctor, lawyer, or teacher. Avoid negative thinking and focus on your goals. When faced with naysayers, stay true to your dreams. Do not let others' negativity deter you. Instead, believe in your ability to achieve your goals through hard work, dedication, and determination.

Set higher boundaries for yourself and be amazed at what you have been missing. Remember, no one is responsible for your downfalls but you. Learn from your struggles and do not let them make you lose hope or vision. Everyone has their story. Mine involves profound loss, which I allowed to hinder my growth for decades. It took me years to pick up the pieces and find my way back. If you face trauma or loss, seek help early. Here are some tips:

1. Seek counseling.
2. Avoid isolating yourself.
3. Accept the impermanence of life.

4. Focus on positive memories.
5. Cherish the bond you shared in your heart.

In conclusion, becoming a better you involves self-awareness, healing, and personal growth. Embrace your journey, learn from your experiences, and do not let negativity hinder your progress.

How To Become A Better Person In The Relationship

"Even though you can only fix you, try to support your spouse/mate in their efforts to change before walking away."

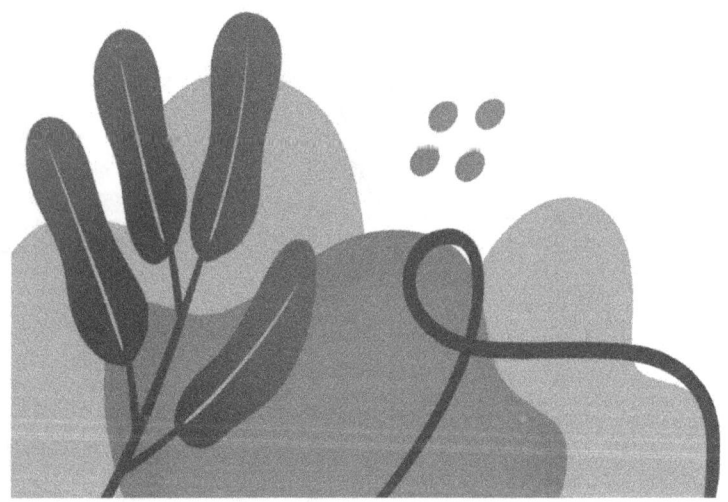

CHAPTER 10

How to Make your Relationship Successful

All relationships, including marriages, have their difficulties, each requiring hard work and commitment. Do not expect it to be easy. It takes dedication, communication, and accepting each other's flaws. We have been with our spouses for years, and it has not always been perfect. There have been many challenges, but we honored our vows and persevered.

There were times we wanted to give up, but we believed in the sanctity of marriage. We turned to our faith, fought against any negative forces, and fought for our union. It was not easy, and yes, it was a struggle. Too often, we give up on our partners/mates too quickly. Before letting someone else benefit from what you have built, try to see the good in your partner and bring out their best.

However, if, after giving all the love and support you have to give, your partner/mate persists in wrongdoing and shows he/she does not care for you or themselves, it may be time to consider ending the relationship. Remember what attracted you to them initially. Often, the goodness you saw is still there; they may have just lost their way. Help them rediscover it.

Even though you can only fix you, try to support your spouse/mate in their efforts to change before walking away. Keep an emotional connection. Address issues promptly and honestly, and do not let them fester. When communicating, do so lovingly, calmly, and safely. Avoid unrealistic expectations, as no partner/mate can meet all your needs. A healthy relationship requires honest and open communication about your needs versus your wants.

Once a problem is resolved, leave it in the past because minor issues can escalate if ignored. Reflect on the early days of your relationship. For instance, when I met my husband, there was an instant connection, and we have worked to keep the flame alive, even as we have aged. It is important to continue dating and spending quality time together.

In today's digital age, it is easy to become distracted by technology. Commit to spending quality time together without the interference of phones or emails. Find shared interests or try new activities together. Keeping a sense of humor and focusing on fun can ease stress and tension.

Communication is not just verbal; body language is important too. Be a good listener, even if you do not always agree. Compromise and respect each other's viewpoints. Remember to forgive and not hold past mistakes against each other.

Sometimes, just listening without responding is enough, especially when your partner/mate needs to vent. Understand that every relationship will have its challenges, including health issues and/or stress. Never take out your frustrations on your spouse/mate. Find healthy outlets for stress, such as hobbies or spiritual practices.

Substance of Building Healthy Relationships

A successful relationship involves handling situations with an open heart and mind. Think before you react and be mindful of the impact of your words. While forgiveness is possible, words can leave lasting impressions. With effort, understanding, and patience, your relationship can thrive through the good and bad times.

Get to Know the Authors

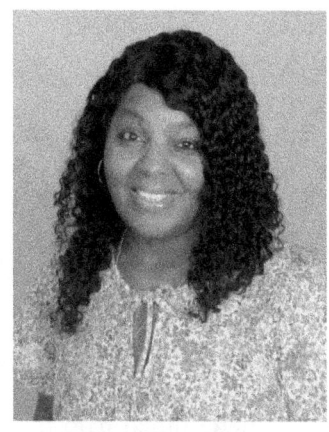

Darlene Mamon

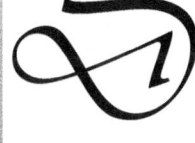arlene is a wife, mother of four, and grandmother to six cherished grandchildren. Born and raised in Chicago by her mother, Leah, and stepfather, Walter Early, Darlene was the third of five children and the only girl. Her childhood in Chicago was marked by tomboyish adventures with her brothers—climbing trees, jumping fences, and excelling at football, much to her brothers' chagrin. Despite the rough and tumble, she was always neatly dressed, with bows in her hair, which puzzled her mother given how quickly she'd get dirty.

Her brothers were tough on her, pushing Darlene to defend herself and stand up against bullies. One brother's advice resonated deeply: never let anyone bully you and be independent. These words became a guiding principle throughout her life, fueling her independent spirit.

At 16, Darlene faced challenges at home that led her to move out, a story she plans to explore in her next book. By 19, she was a mother and went on to have three more children. Her children and grandchildren are her pillars, inspiring her to strive for success and love with all her heart.

Despite cruel words in her past that attempted to undermine her worth, Darlene was determined to prove them wrong. A survivor of three marriages and two divorces, she faced the harshness she was once warned about. Yet, her faith carried her through. She pursued education with vigor, earning her GED and then an Associate Degree in Preschool Education. For 11 years, she led as a head teacher at a local YMCA.

Darlene didn't stop there—she went on to obtain a Bachelor's Degree in Psychology, which led her to a fulfilling role as a Detox Counselor at South Shore Hospital, where she supported individuals striving to overcome drug addiction. Later, she earned a Master's Degree in Mediation and Conflict Resolution, allowing her to aid women in domestic violence situations, drawing from her own experiences as a survivor.

Now residing in Las Vegas, Nevada, with her husband and youngest son, Darlene finds inspiration in the mountains, which stir her soul. She has dedicated 16 years to her career as a Certified Sterile Processing Technician, a role she takes seriously due to its critical impact on patient care in surgeries.

Darlene's creative passion also shines through in her storytelling. As a teacher, she crafted stories for her students, leading to a promise to herself to become an author. By January 2022, she fulfilled that promise, authoring four children's books: "*Children Are A Gift From God,*" "*Busy Busy Tytiana,*" "Tytiana Goes to the Zoo," and the educational "*Adventurous Four,*" a series on African American inventors.

Her artistry extends to crafts, creating 3D pictures that have gained popularity, now sold through her Facebook page, "I Slay MY CRAFT." This success is a testament to her resilience and belief in the power of perseverance and timing. Darlene's life story embodies the ethos that no one else can define your capabilities. With faith at the forefront, she maintains that nothing can impede your path to success.

Contact Darlene Mamon at:
Email: Early_Darlene@yahoo.com

Social Media Accounts:
Facebook: https://bit.ly/New-Wings-Facebook-Group
New Wings Domestic Violence Group

Instagram: https://www.instagram.com/darlenemamon

Get to Know the Authors

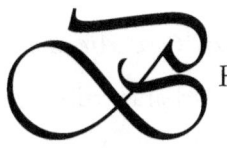arbara Hawkins-Dixon, born on the west side of Chicago, Illinois, is a wife and mother of three. Raised in a single-parent home by her mother, Lucy Hawkins, Barbara was the youngest of ten children. In the late 1960s, her family relocated to the south side of Chicago, where she still resides.

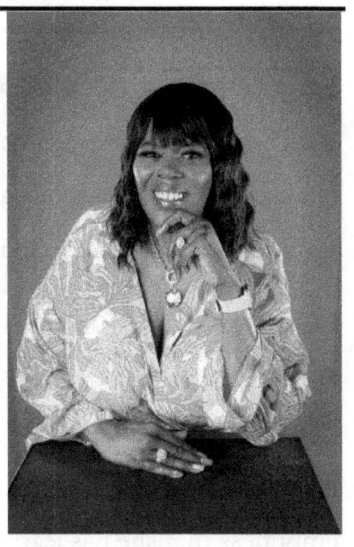

Barbara Hawkins-Dixon

From a young age, Barbara showed an interest in writing but didn't pursue her dream until 2022. This turning point came after a life-altering diagnosis of a brain tumor and subsequent emergency surgery. This experience made her realize she was given a second chance at life, and she was determined to fulfill her dream of becoming a published author.

In 2023, Barbara published her first children's book, "Mama and Daddy, I Want to Help," which became a bestseller on Amazon. She also authored "*Girls Are Made With Sugar and Spice and Everything Nice.*" Barbara attributes her success to her gratitude and faith, continually thanking God for another chance at life.

Despite her achievements, loss and sorrow have marked Barbara's life, including the passing of her mother, two sisters, three brothers, and a cherished nephew. These losses left a profound impact, causing deep sadness and emptiness that she has learned to live with.

Barbara's strength and resilience, inherited from her mother, have been pivotal in her journey. Once broken by family losses and often prioritizing others' feelings over her own, she learned the importance of finding her voice and caring for herself. Her children, grandchildren, and great-grandchildren are her pride and joy, and she loves them unconditionally.

Barbara's career has been diverse, with certifications in medical terminology, criminal justice, advanced childcare, early childhood education, baking, and cake decorating, along with a commercial driving license. She has worked in various roles, including a family advocate for pregnant and parenting teens in Chicago public schools, a teacher's assistant, maintenance and housekeeping in nursing homes, assembly line work, and as a baker and cake decorator, eventually founding L&B Bakery LLC.

Her passion for writing children's books remains strong, and she aspires to become a renowned best-selling author. Barbara believes all things are possible through God, who strengthens her. She emphasizes the importance of building a healthy relationship with oneself before others.

Barbara's most fulfilling career choice was working as a family advocate with Chicago public schools. Identifying with the young pregnant and parenting mothers, she shared her experiences to help them make better decisions. She was deeply invested in helping these young women recognize and leave toxic relationships and abuse. Barbara guided them to resources, helped them continue their education, and often went beyond her duties to ensure they had what they needed.

Barbara's empathy and dedication earned her the respect of her clients. Even though her own teenage parenting experience differed from those of the young mothers she helped, she could relate to and offer genuine concern for them and their children.

There's much more to say about Barbara Hawkins-Dixon, but some stories are reserved for future books.

Contact Barbara Hawkins-Dixon at:
Email: BDixon1931@aol.com

Social Media Accounts:
Facebook:
https://www.facebook.com/barbara.hawkinsdixon
https://bit.ly/Barbara-Hawkins-Dixon-Books

GET TO KNOW THE AUTHORS

www.ingramcontent.com/pod-product-compliance
Lightning Source LLC
Chambersburg PA
CBHW070921160426
43193CB00011B/1548